T0304455

THE HEART OF PRAYER

THE ESSENCE OF MEDITATION SERIES

THE HEART

of

PRAYER

Rupert Spira

SAHAJA

newharbinger
publications

SAHAJA PUBLICATIONS

PO Box 887, Oxford OXI 9PR

www.sahajapublications.com

A co-publication with New Harbinger Publications

5674 Shattuck Ave.

Oakland, CA 94609

United States of America

Distributed in Canada by Raincoast Books

Designed by Rob Bowden

Printed in the United States of America

ISBN 978-1-64848-148-2

Library of Congress Cataloging-in-Publication Data on file with publisher

Our longing for God is God's love for us.

CONTENTS

ACKNOWLEDGEMENTS

I would like to thank all those who have helped with the various aspects of writing, editing, designing and publishing this book. In particular, I would like to thank Lynne Saner, Jacqueline Boyle, Rachel Sopher and Richard John Lewis for their editorial work, and Rob Bowden for preparing the manuscript for publication.

I would also like to express my gratitude to all those who have attended my meetings in person or online, whose deep interest in truth or longing for God elicited the meditations that have been edited for this book.

I would also like to thank everyone at New Harbinger Publications for their continued help and support.

The contemplations in this book are taken from guided meditations that Rupert Spira gave during meetings and retreats from 2020 to 2022. They were originally delivered spontaneously but have been edited for this collection to avoid repetition and to adapt them from the spoken to the written word.

Prayer or meditation takes place in the space between words, although it remains present during the words themselves. Therefore, these contemplations were originally spoken with long silences between sentences or sections, allowing listeners to sink deeply into their being, to which the words point. The meditations in this book have been laid out with numerous breaks between sentences and sections to invite a similarly contemplative approach.

Praise be to God, naked being,
Who wears the universe as its body
And whose name is 'I'.

Praise be to God,
The amness of all selves
Although there are no selves
And the isness of all things
Although there are no things.

Praise be to God,
Who conceals Himself in existence
And reveals Himself as being.

Praise be to God,
Who shrouds Herself in time
And proclaims Herself in eternity.

Praise be to God,
Whose movement is our longing
Whose rest is peace itself.

Praise be to God,
For whom the world is its song
And silence its prayer.

Life is the flight of the alone to the Alone.
PLOTINUS

If God were to confess its experience of itself to us, it might say something like this:

> No one sees me except myself, no one reaches me except myself and no one knows me except myself. I know myself through myself, and I see myself by means of myself alone. No one but I sees myself.
>
> My veil is my oneness since nothing veils me other than myself. I am veiled with my own being. My being is concealed by my oneness without any condition.
>
> No one other than I sees myself. No teacher or student knows me. My teacher is me, my student is me, my message is me and my word is me.
>
> I sent myself from myself through myself to myself. There is no intermediary or means other than me. There is no

difference between the sender, that which is sent and the one to whom it is sent. The very existence of the sacred teaching is my existence. There is no existence to any other who could pass away, or have a name or be named.*

I, infinite, aware being, eternally am.

I am your longing and I am your love; I am your sorrow and I am your joy.

As being, I am hidden; as existence, I am manifest.

It is my being that shines as existence in the world.

If you know your being as my being, you will see the world in myself, as myself.

Just as a screen assumes the form of a landscape without ever ceasing to be itself, thus veiling itself with itself, so I, infinite, aware being, appear to myself as the world without ever being, becoming or knowing anything other than myself.

Just as for one person the landscape in a movie veils the screen and for another it shines with it, so for one the world

* My first-person rendering of Awḥad al-din Balyani, *Know Yourself*, translated by Cecilia Twinch (Beshara Publications, 2011).

veils my being whilst for another it shines as my being. I conceal myself from myself and reveal myself to myself.

You are my veil but I am your reality.

Before anything in the world says anything about itself, it announces my presence. It shines with my being. Everything celebrates me. I overflow within myself in the form of the world.

When I hold up a mirror, my beauty appears as the world. I see the world as my face. When I put away the mirror, I abide as I am.

Make your heart wide enough to contain me and make your actions loving enough to express me.

Turn towards me and I will take you into myself.

CHAPTER I

OUR BEING IS GOD'S BEING

I am silently lost in God.
SAINT CATHERINE OF GENOA

W hat is God?

'I am', before the words 'I am'.

I would like to remain silent here but the written word does not permit.

'I am' is God's confession in our hearts.

Abiding as 'I am' is what God is; abiding as 'I am' is what a person does.

Whatever God is, God must be whole, perfect, complete. From the point of view of the whole, there are no parts. Having no parts, God only knows itself.

No world, no person, no thing. No here or there, before or after, creation or destruction, self or other. No time or space, no thought, no feeling, no body.

This absence of anything other than itself is love.

God knows itself simply by being itself. Its knowing itself is its loving itself.

And what is prayer?

Again, I would like to remain silent, for silence is the closest we come to God before losing ourself in that.

Prayer is simply to remain as the 'I am' before the words 'I am'.

To abide as that. Simply to be.

If this is clear to you, not just philosophically but experientially, read no further. If not, let me elaborate.

*   *   *

To understand what prayer is, it is necessary to understand what the term 'God' refers to. To understand what is meant by God, it is necessary to know what one's self is. Our understanding of God, and thus our understanding of prayer, depends upon our understanding of our self.

As individuals we look at the universe and wonder where it came from. We presume that whatever creates the universe must precede and transcend it. Hence, the conventional idea of a creator God that lies beyond the world, at an infinite distance from ourself, arises as a result of the belief in ourself as an individual. Thus, the trinity of the individual, world and God arises, each an inevitable consequence of the individual's point of view.

Believing God to be the creator of the world and ourself, we then enter into a devotional relationship with it. We could say that the highest state of the individual is to enter into a relationship of devotion to this creator God, surrendering its will to the will of God. This relationship, which is enshrined in much of the world's great religious literature, places the individual in the right relationship to God – one of devotion, adoration, thanksgiving, praise and surrender.

* * *

This path of devotion and surrender gradually purifies and attenuates the individual until the question arises, 'If God's being is infinite, how can there be room for an individual being within it?'

The existence of numerous finite beings would displace a part of infinite being and infinite being would no longer be infinite. God would no longer be God.

3

We come to understand that there is no room for the finite in the infinite.

The individual is not a finite being that exists at a vast distance from infinite being but is an apparent limitation of God's infinite being, the only being there is.

The individual does not surrender; it is surrendered.

Just as there are not numerous physical spaces in the world – one for each building – but one infinite and indivisible space, temporarily enclosed by numerous buildings yet never modified or divided by them, so there are not numerous beings.

There is one being, God's being, temporarily clothed in thoughts and perceptions, seeming to become a temporary, finite self but never actually ceasing to be itself. A human being is God's being temporarily clothed in human attributes. God's being is a human being divested of its qualities.

In prayer, we travel inwards through the layers of experience – thinking, feeling, sensing, perceiving, acting and relating – until we come to our essential, irreducible being. Divested of the qualities that our self derives from the content of experience, it stands revealed as God's infinite being.

The seventeenth-century French monk Brother Lawrence said, 'I removed from my mind everything that was capable of spoiling my communion with God'.* When everything that can be taken from us is removed, all that remains is God's being, and we are that. That is the practice of the presence of God.

Prayer is to understand and feel that the only being in us is God's being, and to abide as that.

Brother Lawrence continues, 'I just make it my business to persevere in the practice of the presence of God. My soul has a constant silent, secret communion with God.' This communion with God is simply remaining with being, *as* being, which lies behind and in the midst of all experience.

There is one being from which everyone and everything derives its apparently independent existence. The infinite appears as the finite without ever ceasing to be itself.

* * *

Existence is being in motion; being is existence at rest.

---

* *The Practice of the Presence of God: The Original 17th Century Letters and Conversations of Brother Lawrence* (Xulon Press, 2007).

Prior to the emergence of things, being is unmanifest. Thus, it is empty, formless, transparent, silent, still.

Prior to the emergence of things, being has nothing in itself other than itself with which it could be divided. Thus, it is indivisible.

Having nothing in itself other than itself, being has no finite qualities with which it could be limited. Thus, it is infinite.

Being shares none of the qualities of ourself as a person, although it is the very essence of ourself and is all there is to ourself, just as a screen shares none of the qualities of the movie and is, at the same time, its essence and reality. Thus, being is impersonal and yet utterly intimate.

Intimate, impersonal, indivisible, infinite being, God's being.

In this understanding, the distinction between the devotee and God gradually diminishes until there is no difference between them. In the absence of any distinction between the one who prays and the one that is prayed to, the devotee and the beloved come closer until there is a great recognition: our being is God's being.

There is no room for an individual in this understanding. There is just God's infinite being and we are that. That is the ultimate surrender.

*   *   *

The individual and God cannot unite, for they were never separate to begin with. As a concession to the apparent individual, what is traditionally referred to as 'union with God' is the revelation of our prior unity. But not even that, for there was never a time when there was a being apart from God's being, either to be separate or unified.

Infinite being knows nothing of separation or union. It is only from the perspective of the apparently separate self that there is separation from God and union with God. There are not two beings, let alone innumerable beings, either to be separate from or united with one another. There is just intimate, impersonal, indivisible, infinite being.

This utter absence of otherness is the experience of love. Thus, love is not a relationship but the absence of relationship, the collapse of the belief and feeling of self and other, individual and God.

This is what the Sufi mystic Jalaluddin Rumi meant when he said, 'In the existence of your love, I become non-existent. This non-existence linked to you is better than anything I ever found in existence.'* In other words, love is God's nature; it is the prior condition of all relationship.

God clothes itself in name and form and appears as the universe. When God undresses, it reveals itself as being. Clothing itself in name and form is the activity of creation; undressing is prayer.

* * *

Our being is not *our* being. It is simply *being*, God's being. Being does not belong to us as a person any more than the space in a room belongs to its four walls. The space was not created when the house was built. The space that seems to be *in* the room is in the same condition it was in before the house was built.

Likewise, God's being in us, as us, is in the same condition now as it was before each of us seems, as a person, to have

* Jalaluddin Rumi, 'I Am Yours', as translated by Fereydoun Kia, in *The Love Poems of Rumi*, Deepak Chopra, ed. (Harmony, 1998).

been born. Nothing ever happens to being. It is coloured by human experience but never conditioned by it.

Just as the space in the room remains in the same pristine condition irrespective of what happens within it, so being remains in the same condition irrespective of whatever we experience. Being is always in the same innocent, ageless, peaceful condition.

Similarly, when the room's walls are taken down, nothing happens to the space. It does not suddenly reunite with the larger space of the universe, because it was never separate from it to begin with. The space simply remains as it always is. It isn't relieved of a limitation, for it was never limited in the first place. There are no individual spaces in the universe either to be separate from or united with the space of the universe. There is always only one space.

Likewise, when this body dies, nothing happens to being. It does not suddenly reunite with God's being, because it was never separate from it to begin with. It does not lose its limitations, for it never acquired any to begin with. It just appeared to be limited from the localised perspective of a finite mind.

To speak of separation and union, distance and closeness, forgetting and remembering is a compassionate concession to the separate self. From its perspective, there seems to be separation and union, distance and closeness, forgetting and remembering. God knows nothing of such things, although all such knowledge is a refraction of God's knowledge of itself.

Being eternally is. Its condition never changes. Being is unborn, without change or death.

*   *   *

One of the principal practices of the great religious and spiritual traditions could be summed up in the Sufi saying, 'Die before you die'. Die in this life as an apparently separate self. Recognise that your being, having lost the finite qualities that it borrows from the content of experience, stands revealed as utterly intimate, yet impersonal, infinite being.

That is the death of the apparently separate self. Our own being is revealed as God's being, and our journey to God comes to an end in that recognition. Then the never-ending journey in God begins, in which the mind, body and world are progressively outshone in God's presence. Our thoughts, feelings, activities and relationships are gradually aligned with this new understanding and become the means by which it is brought into the world and shared with humanity.

There is no great union with God after death. For there to be a union with God in the future, we would have to first stand as a separate being. Union implies separation. There are not two beings – a separate being and God's being – that are now separate and will one day unite. There is just God's being, veiling itself from itself by clothing itself in human experience and then divesting itself of that human experience and recognising itself as it is.

There is concealing and revealing, but never separation or union. Separation and union belong to a preliminary stage of understanding that credits the separate self with its own independent existence. For that one, the teaching says, 'Behave well, and when you die you will unite with God', but at a deeper level the teaching doesn't credit the individual with their own independent existence.

It is a misunderstanding to set oneself up as a being apart from God's being. To say, 'I am God' is not blasphemous, although one should never say such a thing. What is blasphemous is to say, 'I am a person'. In doing so, we set ourself up as a being apart from God's being. If we were separate from God's being, there would be two or more beings, and thus God's being would not be infinite and God would not be God. *That* is blasphemy. Likewise, to see another as other is to assert that there are two beings, which is to deny God's being.

When we look inside ourself we find thoughts, images, feelings and sensations, but if we travel further back through these layers, we find only God's being. When pure being becomes mixed with thoughts and feelings, it acquires a limit and seems to become a person. Even then, it is still only God's infinite being, albeit clothed in personal experience.

Ultimately, there is no separate self either to be separate from or united with God. There is only God's being, concealing itself in human experience and revealing itself. To die before we die means to go deeply into ourself, through the layers of personal experience, until we get to simply being, the raw experience 'I am'. That experience is utterly intimate – it is our very self – but is impersonal and unlimited. It is God's being.

Being eternally is. I eternally am.

*   *   *

What becomes of our devotion when the devotee and the beloved are recognised to be the same? Just as when attention is relieved of its object, it subsides into its source of pure awareness, so when the one who is devoted and the one to whom they are devoted are recognised as one and the same, devotion loses its direction, its dynamism, and sinks back into the objectless love from which it arose.

'Lord, Thou art the love with which I love Thee.'*

In prayer, notice any impulse to move away from simply being towards someone or something objective. To move away from being towards an object of experience is the residue of an old habit of seeking God outside ourself. But in order to seek God outside ourself, we must first set ourself up as a self apart from God's being, and, in doing so, we strengthen the feeling of separation, thereby alienating ourself from God.

God lies at the source of our longing and can never be an object of it. Let any impulse to move away from simply being come to rest in this understanding. There is no room for effort in prayer, for effort would always be from what is to what is not yet.

What seems from the point of view of the individual to be an effort that it makes towards God is, in fact, the gravitational pull of God's being acting on the apparent individual.

* Attributed to a sixteenth-century Italian monk.

This gravitational pull of God's being on its own contracted form – the individual – is grace.

Every individual's desire for happiness, peace, love, justice, understanding, compassion or beauty is really the individual's response to the pull of grace that they feel in their heart.

Our longing for God is God's love for us. It is the pull of our being inviting us to return from the adventure of experience to the sanctuary of the heart, to return home.

Our longing never finds what it is looking for; it comes to rest in it.

Prayer is not a movement from ourself towards God. It is a divesting of ourself of all the qualities we seem to have acquired from experience, and the subsequent revelation of our being as God's infinite being.

In this understanding, effort loses its dynamism and gives way to surrender.

Our longing is gradually divested of its dynamism and subsides into the love from which it arose. It finds at its source what it previously sought as its destiny.

There is no longer room for a movement from the individual towards God. Any residual becoming comes to an end. The silence that remains is our prayer.

*   *   *

In prayer, we sink deeply into simply being. As we abide as that, our being is divested, usually gradually but occasionally suddenly, of the limitations that it acquires from human experience and stands revealed as God's infinite being.

Infinite being is not something that is known objectively. It is what remains when nothing is known. It could be called divine ignorance, the 'cloud of unknowing' that is darkness to the mind but light to the heart.

In the Bhagavad Gita it says, 'What is known by the mind is unknown to God, and what is known by God is unknown to the mind'.* The mind refracts reality, God's being, making it appear as a multiplicity and diversity of objects and selves. Thus, the mind superimposes its own limitations onto the reality it perceives, causing it to appear in a way that is consistent with and an expression of its own limitations. Thus, just as one cannot see white snow

* The Bhagavad Gita, 2:69.

through orange-tinted glasses, the mind cannot know reality as it essentially is, although everything that it knows is an appearance of it.

The infinite can only know the infinite. Therefore, God's being cannot know anything finite directly. To know the finite, the infinite must contract into a finite mind from whose perspective it perceives itself as the multiplicity and diversity of the world.

Prayer is the reversal of this process – the individual loses the limitations that it acquires from experience and stands revealed as infinite being. As it loses its limitations, so the world loses the limitations that the finite mind imposed on it and stands revealed as the same infinite being. What we essentially are and what the world essentially is are the same.

Prayer is to abide in the empty sanctuary of the heart – to know nothing, be nothing, seek nothing. In prayer, we do not allow our being to become personalised by experience. Being is utterly intimate, closer than close and, at the same time, impersonal and infinite.

We allow our self to be as impersonal as God, and we allow God to be as intimate as our self.

* * *

Infinite being is that from which everything derives its apparently independent existence. Thought divides it into names and perception refracts it into forms. As such, the activities of thought and perception fragment God's infinite being, making it appear as a multiplicity and diversity of objects and selves.

None of these objects and selves are such in their own right. They are modulations of the one ever-present reality, God's being.

In the words of the Sufi mystic Awhad al-din Balyani, 'He was described as every day in a different configuration when there was no "thing" other than Him. And He is now as He has always been, since in reality what is other than Him has no being. Just as in eternity-without-beginning and time-lessness, He was every day in a different configuration when no thing existed, so He is now as He has always been, although there is no thing or day, just as there has been from all eternity no thing or day. The existence of the creatures and their non-existence are the same.'*

* From Awhad al-din Balyani, *Know Yourself*, translated by Cecilia Twinch (Beshara Publications, 2011).

Creation and destruction only seem to be real from the limited perspective of the individual. However, nothing is created; nothing is destroyed. No person or thing has its own independent existence. All borrow their apparent existence from that which truly is: the being that shines in our experience as the amness of our self and in the world as the isness of things.

Nothing – no thing – exists. Only God truly is.

*   *   *

Be sensitive to any impulse to leave this 'cloud of unknowing' in favour of the known. The sanctuary of the heart is dark. Nothing can be seen or known there, nothing sought. Let the residue of becoming dissolve in being.

From the individual's perspective, prayer is a movement of itself towards God. In reality, prayer is emptying ourself of ourself, the subsidence of ourself in God's being.

When our being is divested of all the limited qualities that it acquires from experience, it stands revealed as infinite being. As the thirteenth-century German mystic Meister Eckhart said, 'To be empty of things is to be full of God. The very best attainment in life is to remain still and let God act and speak in you. But God is not found in the soul by adding anything but by a process of subtraction.'*

As such, forgetfulness of self is remembrance of God. This self-forgetting is the essence of prayer. We could equally say that the remembrance of self – infinite, impersonal being – is the ultimate prayer.

Emptiness of self is the fullness of God.

To know something other than God one must set oneself up as a separate subject of experience, a being apart from God. That is, things are only things from the individual's point of view. Thus, knowledge of things is said to veil God's presence. But for one who knows their being as God's being, the world loses its concealing power and becomes a revealing power. It shines with its reality, God's presence.

With your mind know ten thousand things, but with your heart feel only one reality.

*   *   *

* *Meister Eckhart, the Essential Sermons, Commentaries, Treatises, and Defense*, translated and edited by Edmund Colledge and Bernard McGinn (Paulist Press, 1981).

Once we have understood that our being is God's being, we can return to the devotional literature contained in the great religious and spiritual traditions and understand that, though written in conventional dualistic language, it shines with this same understanding.

O my Lord, my whole being is Your self, and this mind which has been given to me is Your consort.

The life-force, breath and energy which You have given me are Your attendants.

My body is the temple in which I worship You.

Whatever I eat or wear or do is all part of the worship which I keep on performing at this temple.

Even when this body goes to sleep at night, I feel I am in union with You.

Whenever I walk, I feel I am going on pilgrimage to You.

Whatever I speak is all in praise of You.

So whatever I do in this world in any way is all aimed at You.

In fact, there is no duality in this life of union with Your self.*

---

* A prayer given to Dr. Francis Roles in 1977 by Shantananda Saraswati, the late Shankaracharya of the north of India.

CHAPTER 2

THE DIVINE NAME

There is only one ego, only one selfhood, the I Am that I Am,
that I in the midst of us, the divine selfhood of you and me.
JOEL GOLDSMITH

I magine the universe billions of years ago, before there were any objects or planets within it – a vast, empty physical space. Now imagine adding the quality of knowing or awareness to it so that the universe is now a vast, empty, *aware* physical space.

What are the qualities of this space? We could say it is un-limited or infinite, although that wouldn't be quite right, as there is not yet anything limited or finite inside it with which to contrast it.

If we were to ask this space, 'What is your name?', it would answer, 'I', because 'I' is the name that anything that knows itself gives to itself. Likewise, the reason why each of us refers to our self as 'I' is because we *know* our self.

If we were to now ask this space, 'What is the first thing you can say for certain about yourself?', it would respond, 'I am'. 'I am' refers to its primary knowledge of itself.

Now imagine we were to take a sample of this space, put it in a jar and fast-forward thirteen billion years to today. It is now populated with planets, objects, buildings, people, animals and so on.

If we were again to ask this space, which now seems to be contained within the four walls of a room, to describe itself, it would look around and respond, 'I am small' or 'I am large'; 'I am dark' or 'I am light'; 'I am cluttered' or 'I am empty'. However, in each case the space is not describing itself; it is describing the qualities it appears to derive from the walls within which it seems to be contained or from the objects within it.

But what about the space itself? Imagine we were to take a sample of the space in the room and compare it with the sample we took before there were any planets or objects. Would there be any difference between the two?

No, they would be identical! The space inside the room is the same infinite, unlimited, unqualified space that it was before anything came into existence.

Now imagine removing the space-like quality from this compound of space and awareness, so it is no longer a vast, aware, physical space but simply *aware being*. We cannot even call it vast, for in the absence of space it is not extended in any dimension, either of time or space. That aware being is our self.

Just as the space of a room seems to be qualified by its four walls but is, in fact, unqualified and unlimited, so our apparently finite being is not qualified by or limited to the content of experience.

Just as there are no limited physical spaces in the universe but only one infinite space, so there are no limited beings or individual selves. There is just one unlimited, infinite being, God's being.

The finite self that we seem to be is God's being, the only being there is, temporarily qualified by, and seemingly limited to, the content of experience.

*   *   *

Imagine we were to ask the being that we essentially are, God's being, what it would call itself if it were to give itself a name. It would respond, 'I', for 'I' is the name that whatever knows itself gives to itself.

'I' is God's name in each of us.

Jane, Sophie, Peter and John are the names we give to each other, but 'I' is the name we give to our self. 'I' refers to the subjective experience of simply being or being aware, before it is qualified by experience.

Our knowledge of our self is God's knowledge of itself.

This is what the Sufis mean when they say, 'I searched for myself and found only God. I searched for God and found only myself.'

'I' is the constant factor in all changing experience, like the invisible thread upon which the beads of a necklace are strung. Without it, there would just be a hundred disconnected beads. It is the thread that confers integrity and singularity upon the necklace.

'I' is the hidden thread that runs throughout our life. Without it, experience would be a chaos of thoughts, images and feelings. Experience is always one thing, not ten thousand things. Experience borrows its oneness from the singularity of 'I'.

No matter what the content of experience, the sense of 'I', the feeling of being, pervades it, shining brightly like a beacon in its midst.

'I' is the first form of God, the first utterance. Keep the name 'I' sacred. Do not allow it to become tarnished by experience.

If we feel that we are lost in experience, all that is necessary is to sound the divine name, 'I', once in our mind and follow it to that which is named. Like Ariadne's golden thread, it leads directly to the presence of God in our hearts.

Traditionally, church bells would toll to invite people to pause their daily tasks and remember God's presence. Every time we think or speak the name 'I', we should pause and consider it an invitation to turn away from the content of experience in which we were previously involved and come back to God's presence in our heart.

To live a life of prayer means to be in constant communion with being and not allow it to become mixed with or veiled by experience. Meister Eckhart said, 'God is a great underground river that no one can dam up and no one can stop'.* The great river of being flows behind and within all experience, continually changing its name and form but never changing its essence.

* Matthew Fox, *Meditations with Meister Eckhart* (Bear & Company, 1983).

To 'pray without ceasing', as they say in the Orthodox Church, does not mean to be constantly reciting a verbal prayer or repeating a mantra, but to remain continually in touch with this great underground river of being that intimately pervades all experience irrespective of its content.

*   *   *

In all the great religious and spiritual traditions, the one reality, the supreme being, is given numerous names: Brahman, Buddha, the Tao, Consciousness, Being, Shiva, Allah, Spirit, Love, Jehovah. Indeed, God itself is one such name.

However, to name anything, we must first stand apart from that thing and know it from a distance. Therefore, anything we name cannot be our self and cannot, as such, be the name of God, for God is our very own being.

God's true name can only be the name that it would give *itself*. What would God call itself? 'I', for 'I' is the name that that which knows itself gives to itself. Therefore, God's most sacred name is 'I'.

As Meister Eckhart says, 'And so the word "I" denotes God's purity of essence, which is bare in itself, free of alien elements that make it strange and distant'.*

As a concession to the apparently separate self, all of God's names are valid and stand as emblems pointing us in the right direction. However, 'I' is a unique name. It does not point to anything outside our self but points directly to our innermost being, God's infinite being. Thus, the name 'I' is in a different category from all other names and its power is immeasurably greater.

Of all God's names, 'I' is the highest and most sacred, indicating God's subjective knowledge of itself. It is the divine name.

However, 'I' is not only the most sacred name but also the most powerful mantra. A mantra is a sound that has a vibrational frequency that is the condensed essence of the primordial sound that God utters and that later expands as the universe. The mantra is a precipitation of this primordial sound, with a vibrational frequency that acts on the mind in such a way as to return it to its source.

* *The Complete Mystical Works of Meister Eckhart*, translated by Maurice O'C. Walshe (Herder & Herder, 2010).

If we sound the name 'I' and allow it to take us to the *experience* 'I', that is, if 'I' disentangles itself from the content of experience and comes back to itself, it stands divested of all qualification and limitation as the infinite 'I', God's being.

*   *   *

Each of us can say from our own direct experience that 'I am'. And each of us can say for certain that I am because I *know* that I am. The 'I' that knows that I am is the *same* 'I' that I am. In other words, the knowledge 'I am' is our being's knowledge of itself. Therefore, the name 'I' refers not just to being but to being's knowledge of itself, the awareness of being.

Being's awareness of itself is an utterly unique knowledge. Everything else that is known or experienced is known or experienced by something other than itself. A thought is not known by itself; it is known by awareness. A tree is not perceived by itself; it is perceived by awareness. An emotion is not felt by itself; it is felt by awareness. However, being is known *by* itself. Being is, as such, self-knowing or self-aware.

Moreover, everything apart from the awareness of being is known through the faculties of a finite mind, and appears relative to it and in accordance with its qualities. Thus, all knowledge and experience is relative to the finite mind through which it is known and shares its limitations.

However, being knows itself *directly*. Its knowledge of itself is not mediated through or relative to a finite mind. It is, as such, absolute knowledge. The name 'I' refers to that knowledge, to the absolute. We should tremble at the sound of it.

*　　*　　*

Before our being is qualified by the content of experience, it knows no limit in itself. The knowledge 'I am' is infinite being's knowledge of itself.

In the Old Testament, God says to Moses, 'I am that I am'. Later God says, 'Tell the people of Israel, "I am has sent me to you" '.*

God's presence shines in each of us as the experience 'I am'. God is the very being of our being, therefore, our knowledge of our self is God's knowledge of itself. Our experience of our self is God's experience of itself.

It is for this reason that Meister Eckhart said, 'The eye through which I see God is the same eye through which

* The Book of Exodus, 3:14.

God sees me. My eye and God's eye are one eye, one seeing, one knowing, one love.'*

When our being becomes mixed with the content of experience, it seems to acquire its qualities and limitations. Infinite being seems to become a temporary, finite being. 'I am' becomes 'I am this' or 'I am that'. God's being seems to become a human being without ever actually ceasing to be itself.

This amalgam of infinite being with the qualities of experience gives rise to a human being. That is, a human being is God's being clothed in human experience. However, although infinite being is clothed in human experience, it is not qualified by it. Our clothes change the appearance of our body but not its nature.

Likewise, experience changes the *appearance* of our self – not only the body, but our thoughts, feelings, actions and relationships – but it does not change the *nature* of our self, God's being.

In prayer, we do not *become* our naked being. We do not travel from one kind of self to another, one being

* Walshe *op. cit.*

to another. Our being is simply undressed or unveiled. Just as when we undress at night our naked body is revealed, so, in prayer, we are divested of the content of experience and stand revealed as God's naked being.

We are, in fact, always only God's utterly intimate, impersonal being. God's being simply ceases to clothe itself in human experience. It comes back to itself from the adventure of experience, although, in reality, it never really left itself or became anything other than itself.

It conceals itself with itself and reveals itself to itself.

As God's being clothes itself in human experience, it passes out of eternity into time. More accurately, it doesn't pass out of eternity, because there is nothing in God's being other than God's being into which it could pass. Rather, God sees its own eternity as time when it looks at itself through the medium of a finite mind. As such, time is how eternity appears from the perspective of a human being.

The name 'I' is like a portal through which God passes out of eternity into time and seems to become a finite being, and the same portal, traversed in the opposite direction, through which a finite being passes out of time into eternity.

As it passes through that portal, it loses its limited qualities and stands revealed as God's being.

Do not allow yourself to be personalised or limited by experience. No experience has ever qualified, diminished, hurt, changed or aggrandised you. As Meister Eckhart said, 'There is a place in the soul that has never been wounded'.* Our being is in the same condition now as it was before the birth of our body and will remain the same after its death. We are always the same infinite, pristine, self-aware being.

God's being always remains the same perfect, unblemished, indivisible whole, the unqualified 'I am' that shines like a beacon behind and in the midst of all experience, irrespective of its content.

God leaves a trace of itself in each of us as the knowledge 'I' or 'I am'. 'I' or 'I am' is, as such, God's signature in each of our minds. The feeling of being is God's presence in each of our hearts. Thus, 'I' or 'I am' is the divine name, the first form of God.

All that is necessary is to repeat God's name once and listen in the silence that ensues for God's response, 'I am here'.

* Walshe *op. cit.*

Each of our given names is also a sacred name. When we hear our name, we respond, 'Yes'. What happens in the brief pause between the sound of our name and our response? We refer to our self. Not to our thoughts and feelings, or a sensation in the body, but to our self, God's being. As such, all names are the names of God. This is what it means in the Old Testament when God says, 'I have called you by name. You are mine.'*

*   *   *

In prayer or meditation, we sound the name 'I' or 'I am' once in our mind and allow ourself to be drawn into its referent. We simply emphasise the 'I am' aspect of experience.

When most people feel, for instance, 'I am lonely', they ignore the 'I am' and emphasise the loneliness. When tired, they ignore the 'I am' and emphasise the tiredness. When sick, they ignore the 'I am' and emphasise the sickness.

All that is necessary is to soften the focus of our attention from the content of experience and emphasise the 'I am'. As Meister Eckhart said, 'Our whole life ought to be being. So far as our life is being, so far it is in God.'† Or as Brother

* The Book of Isaiah, 43:1.
† Walshe op. cit.

Lawrence said, 'I have abandoned all particular forms of devotion, all prayer techniques. My only prayer practice is attention. I carry on a habitual, silent and secret conversation with God that fills me with overwhelming joy.' *

We allow being to emerge from the background of experience, where it lies unnoticed most of the time, into the foreground, and we allow the content of experience, which occupies our attention most of the time, to subside into the background.

The disentangling of our self from the qualities of experience is the essence of prayer or meditation. In everyday life, experience obscures being; in prayer, being outshines experience.

When my first teacher, Dr. Francis Roles, met Shantananda Saraswati, the Shankaracharya of the north of India, he said it was like seeing a man guarding a candle in the wind. That is a beautiful image of prayer. We do not allow the awareness of being to be extinguished by the awareness of experience.

The experience 'I am' is like a candle in the wind to be guarded carefully.

* *The Practice of the Presence of God: The Best Rule of Holy Life*, edited by Anthony Uyl (Devoted Publishing, 2018).

CHAPTER 3

BE WITHOUT BECOMING

*All that God asks you most pressingly is to go
out of yourself and let God be God in you.*
MEISTER ECKHART

One of the world's greatest spiritual masterpieces, Jalaluddin Rumi's *Mathnawi*, is an outpouring of surrender and praise to God:

Listen to the yearning of the reed, how it sighs with the wound of separation, saying:

'Ever since I was plucked from my reedbed, I have uttered this lament in the hopes that anyone who feels sorrowful or alone will hear my call.

Anyone who has been separated from someone they love will understand my song. Every separation is an echo in the heart of the great separation, every sorrow an invitation to return. Anyone who has been taken from their home longs to go back.

I sing the same song amongst those who are happy and those who are sad. I am a friend to all, and each hears according to their own experience. But few can hear the secret that is hidden within my music, for my music cannot be heard with the ears. It can only be heard with the heart.

It is love's fire that breathes in me, not wind. If you do not know this love, you do not know yourself. It is the taste of love that is distilled into wine. If you have not tasted this wine, you have never really been drunk.

My music is a friend to all those who long for the wound of separation to be healed. My poignancy intensifies their longing. My sweetness offers them respite.

Allow my music to live in your heart. In it, you will hear your longing for God and, at the same time, God's love for you.'*

*　　*　　*

When I first heard Rumi's poetry, a childhood intuition was re-awakened in me: the entire universe is a dream in God's mind, made only of God, known only by God, and our purpose as individuals is to explore and

---

* My rendition of the beginning of Jalaluddin Rumi's epic poem *Mathnawi*.

recognise reality as that, and to live and celebrate it to the best of our ability.

Little did I realise that an eternal truth had formulated itself in my mind: surrender and praise are the natural state of the individual and is that to which all our lives are tending, whether we realise it or not.

Someone once asked Rumi, 'What is a Sufi?' His reply: 'One with a broken heart'. A broken heart is the state of one who feels an existential longing for something, they know not what, which cannot be requited or fulfilled by anyone or anything in this world, although anyone we love is the face of that one.

But why this longing? What is its source and why do we all feel it?

When we look inside for it, we often find an emptiness, an impulse of seeking or resisting, which is so uncomfortable that we flee from it into objects, substances, activities and relationships. But when the object subsides, the substance wears off or the activity or relationship comes to an end, the emptiness bubbles up again. Eventually, through exhaustion or frustration, we begin to intuit that nothing objective could ever satisfy this longing.

What is it that we long for? Any attempt to name it falls short. Even to call it God is to give it a name and is, as such, an attempt to bring it within the compass of the finite mind. In doing so, we subtly avoid it. By bringing the object of our longing within its own sphere of knowledge, the mind perpetuates itself, thereby avoiding the one thing necessary: its surrender.

Although I refer many times to that for which we all deeply long as God, it would be better to leave it unnamed, for without a name it cannot be grasped by the mind or found in any known direction.

Once we give a name to that for which we long, we can approach it, move towards it. We have reduced it to an image. Even to conceive the object of our search as God is to objectify it. Although God is the subtlest of all objects in which we seek relief from sorrow, dissatisfaction or loneliness, eventually we must have the courage and clarity to recognise that even this is a subtle avoidance.

It is in this context that Meister Eckhart said, 'I pray to God to rid me of God'.* To the church, this was the ultimate

* Sermon 87, 'Blessed Are the Poor in Spirit', as translated by Oliver Davies in *Selected Writings* (Penguin, 1995).

blasphemy, but for one who understands, it was a prayer that the last vestige of objectivity which separated his being from God's being be removed so that he might recognise his own being as God's being.

* * *

If we are approaching someone or something, even if that thing is the ultimate object of our longing – God, enlightenment, salvation and so on – we stand apart from it as a separate subject of experience. As such, our movement or approach is a movement of separation.

To seek God is to deny God.

The lover does not unite with the beloved. It dies in the beloved.

> The One remains, the many change and pass;
> Heaven's light forever shines, Earth's shadows fly;
> Life, like a dome of many-coloured glass,
> Stains the white radiance of Eternity,
> Until Death tramples it to fragments. – Die,
> If thou wouldst be with that which thou dost seek.*

* Percy Bysshe Shelley, from 'Adonais' (1821).

If the object of our longing remains nameless and formless, we cannot go towards it. We remain without direction, impulse or becoming – open, empty and available.

Just as it is not possible to have a subject without an object, or an object without a subject, so it is not possible to have a beloved without a lover or a lover without a beloved. Perhaps the most difficult thing for one on the path of love or devotion is to recognise that by maintaining the object of their devotion they are maintaining their self as a separate subject of experience and ultimately, as such, denying their beloved.

Any impulse to move away from our current experience perpetuates the one who is dissatisfied, the separate self that we believe and feel ourself to be. For this reason, Rumi said, 'Don't run away from grief. Look for the remedy inside the pain itself, because the rose came from the thorn and the ruby came from the stone.'*

It is not feelings themselves that are problematic but our turning away from them. In the way of surrender, we turn towards that from which we previously turned away. We embrace that which is most distasteful to us. First we

* Jalaluddin Rumi, from 'Poem', in *The Essential Rumi*, translated by Coleman Barks (HarperOne, 2004).

surrender our resistance, then we surrender the one who resists, then we surrender the surrendering. As a result, right at the very heart of the experience, we find the peace and joy we previously sought by avoiding it.

* * *

Many of us recognise that our longing or dissatisfaction cannot be satisfied by objects, substances, activities and relationships. Consequently, we approach a religious or spiritual tradition. However, eventually we realise that even our religious or spiritual tradition is a subtle object, more refined than the objects in which we previously sought peace and happiness, yet still something objective to which we direct our attention or offer our love.

Ultimately, we must let go of our devotion to our teachers, teachings, practices and traditions. To this end, sometimes a teacher may banish or ignore a student, or do or say something that severs a connection which, at a deeper level, doesn't seem to make sense but is a kind of impersonal act of grace, freeing us from any last attachments.

Feel any impulse to invest your identity in anyone or anything, to reach away from yourself towards God or enlightenment, however refined or noble that impulse might be. Allow this impulse to come to rest in understanding and love.

Allow becoming to subside in being.

*   *   *

Be without becoming.

In being without becoming, there is no movement of our self, no dynamism, tension, attention or devotion. We do not go towards that for which we long; we sink into it. This sinking takes place on the vertical dimension of being, not the horizontal dimension of becoming. It takes place in a directionless direction that cannot be known by the mind.

As Rumi said, 'Live in silence. Flow down and down in always widening rings of being.'* As we sink into being, our being is divested of the qualities that it derives from the content of experience and stands revealed as utterly intimate, yet impersonal, infinite being.

The side-effect of this sinking into the depths of being is the release of tension in the body and agitation in the mind.

* Jalaluddin Rumi, 'A Community of the Spirit', *Selected Poems*, translated by Coleman Barks (Penguin, 2004).

The mind and body come to rest as an inevitable consequence of this self-abidance.

Our suffering is relieved of its seeking and is revealed as peace and happiness. Our longing is relieved of its dynamism and is revealed as love.

We do not really long for love. Our longing is already that love, albeit thinly veiled by the belief that there is something other than God's presence.

Longing is the veiling of love; love is the subsidence of longing.

*　　*　　*

In the Sufi tradition, every sorrow is an echo in our heart of the great separation from which everyone longs to be healed. The Sufi is one who turns towards that sorrow and embraces it. 'The hurt that we embrace becomes joy. Gather it into your arms, where it can be transformed.'* For the Sufi, grief, sorrow and despair are not considered negative emotions or experiences to be avoided or transformed; they are considered invitations that God sends directly to our hearts, the voice of God calling us home.

* Attributed to Jalaluddin Rumi.

Through misunderstanding, we believe that it is we, as a person, who pray to God, but there is no such person. The person is an imaginary limit, self-assumed by the only one who truly is.

Ultimately, there are no human beings. There is just infinite being, God's being, clothed in human experience, without ever ceasing to be itself or becoming anything other than itself. As such, every experience of sorrow, grief or loss is the gravitational pull of God's presence in our heart calling us back into itself.

Our longing for God is God's love for us.

It is not we who pray to God but God who prays to us:

> Where have you been, my love?
> Come back to Me.
> I am closer to you than your breath.
> I am more intimate than your deepest feeling.
> I am the self of your self.
> I am the being of your being.
> I am the 'I am' in you.
> I cannot be found but I am never lost.
> I cannot be known but am never not known.
> Turn towards Me and I will take you into Myself.
> Come back, come back, come back.

*   *   *

Let all becoming come to rest in being.

Let your longing come to rest in love.

Desire is the movement of our longing towards an object, which leads to pleasure. Prayer or meditation is the subsidence of our longing in the subject, which leads to peace and joy.

Any expectation implies the absence of that which is expected. How can that which truly is be absent? That which truly is *is* and shines in us as the knowledge 'I am'. Our expectation does not arise on account of its absence; our expectation *creates* its apparent absence.

If we expect some experience to appear, then eventually it may appear, but even if it does, it would, by definition, eventually disappear, because everything that appears must disappear. Therefore, its appearance could not possibly lead to God's presence and the peace and quiet joy that accompany it.

All our sorrow exists in the discrepancy between what we have and what we want. When what we have and what we want converge, our innate peace and joy shine. When what we have and what we want diverge, our innate peace and joy are veiled.

Nothing needs to change. Our thoughts do not need to be stilled; our emotions do not need to be changed; our circumstances do not need to be improved. There is nothing to become, acquire, achieve or know. We are already that for which we long. We are not seeking happiness. It is happiness which seeks us.

We do not need to *become* enlightened. We are already the light of the self, the light of pure being. Our search for God is the veiling of God's being. To search for God is to set oneself up as a being apart from God's being, and that is blasphemy.

*   *   *

There is no aspect of our experience that is not completely saturated with being. If I am depressed, I am present there. If I am in love, I am present there. If I am sick, tired or lonely, I am present there. If I am meditating, walking or drinking tea, I am present there. Whatever I am thinking, feeling, sensing or perceiving, I am present there.

No experience has the capacity to veil our being unless we give it permission to do so, in which case it will seem to do so.

As soon as we withdraw that permission, the experience which once seemed to veil our being will now shine with it.

It is not the landscape in the movie that veils the screen. It is our *belief* that the landscape is a real landscape that *seems* to make the screen invisible. When we remember that the landscape is part of the movie, the screen, which once seemed to be veiled by it, now shines with it. The screen was not veiled by the landscape; it was veiled by our belief.

Likewise, it is not experience itself that veils being; it is *belief* that seems to veil it. Once this is clear, we cease having an agenda with the content of experience, and being emerges from the background of experience and now shines in the foreground.

Just as the space of a room is the vast space of the universe temporarily qualified by its four walls, so our being is God's being temporarily coloured by the qualities of experience but never actually ceasing to be itself. It never becomes anything other than itself. It pervades the body but is not generated by, limited to or contained within it.

Thought alone confers limitations on being and imagines a temporary, finite, separate being – a being which owes its reality to infinite being but derives its limitations from the content of experience. This mixture of God's infinite being with the limitations or qualities of experience, creates the temporary, finite, separate self around whom most people's lives revolve, on behalf of whom most of their thoughts and feelings arise, and in whose service their activities and relationships are undertaken.

Ask yourself, 'What is the nature of my being after it has been divested of all the qualities it borrows from experience?' Don't answer that question with a word. The question is an invitation to take us deeply into the experience of simply being and taste its nature.

The fact of simply being is whole, perfect and complete, needing nothing, wanting nothing and lacking nothing. Divested of the qualities that our essential being borrows from the content of experience, being has no limits or divisions within itself.

It is utterly intimate or innermost but, at the same time, unlimited or infinite. It is the essence of ourself as a person but is not itself personal: intimate, indivisible, infinite, impersonal being, God's being, which shines in our experience as our very own self.

We cannot become what we already are through effort, practice or discipline, nor can we cease being what we eternally are through negligence or error. We overlook our self and remember our self. We become lost in the content of experience, and then we return to and recognise our self.

* * *

If we were to ask being, 'What is your experience of yourself?', the first thing it would say, if it could speak, would be, 'I am'. The knowledge 'I am' is God's signature in our hearts. When we allow our being to be qualified by experience, 'I am' becomes, 'I am this' or 'I am that'. God's infinite being seems to become a temporary, finite self or ego.

If we were to ask being to tell us more about itself, it would say, 'I find nothing in myself other than myself with which I could be disturbed or distracted. Thus, my nature is peace. In my own experience of myself, there is just the fullness of myself. There is no sorrow. I am eternally at peace and unconditionally fulfilled.'

If we look outside ourself at the world, we find that whatever exists – an atom, a tree, a building, a planet – is pervaded by and has its existence in being. It is not possible for something to exist outside being any more than a physical object can exist outside space. In what medium would the object exist if it existed outside space? In what medium would anything exist if it existed outside being? Whatever might exist outside being would not *be*.

The being that shines in each of us as the amness of our self is the same being that shines in the world as the isness of things. Separate, limited objects only seem to exist from the point of view of a separate, limited self or being. In reality, the apparently separate, inside self and the apparently separate object, other or world are two aspects of the same inseparable, indivisible whole, whose nature is pure being.

There is no otherness or separation in being. If we were to ask being, 'What is your experience of yourself?', it would say, 'I never know anything other than myself'. As Balyani said, 'Other than Him is Him without otherness'.* As such, the nature of being is love.

All the great religious and spiritual traditions draw their knowledge from this single understanding: peace and happiness are the nature of our being and we share our being with everyone and everything. This understanding is not only the direct path to the peace and happiness for which all people long above all else, but is also the foundation for

* Twinch *op. cit.*

the resolution of conflicts between individuals, communities and nations. It must also be the basis for the restoration of a harmonious relationship with the planet.

In time, this understanding sinks more deeply into us. It doesn't just pervade our minds but floods our hearts. It permeates the body and flows out into the world.

This is the process that is referred to in the Christian tradition as the Transfiguration, the gradual pervading of everything with the light of pure being, and the eventual transfiguring of everything into that. It is the outshining of all experience in God's being.

*   *   *

Whatever exists in the world *is*. A tree *is*. A mountain *is*. An atom *is*. Indeed, the world *is*. As such, isness or being is the common factor in all things and cannot, therefore, be limited to, or share the qualities of, any particular thing.

Just as being is impersonal and yet the very essence of the person, so being is not in the world but is the essence of it. Just as experience temporarily colours being on the inside, so existence temporarily colours being on the outside.

'Existence', from the Latin *ex sistere*, means 'to stand out from', implying that all existent things stand out from the background of infinite being. In fact, nothing really stands out from being, for if anything did, that in which it stood or existed would not be. Everything moves, lives and has its existence in being. The same being that shines as the essence of our self on the inside shines as the essence of all things on the outside. Subjectively, being is experienced as the amness of our self, and objectively as the isness of things.

Just as it is not necessary to turn away from the content of experience, but rather to soften the focus of our attention from its content and allow being to be magnified in our experience, so it is not necessary to turn away from the world. We simply allow it to become increasingly transparent to its essence, pure being. As we do so, the world which once seemed to conceal its reality now shines with it.

Only being *is*, shining as the amness of our self and the isness of things.

Anything that exists emerges within being, but being never passes out of itself into existence. It simply colours itself with its own activity. When being colours itself in the form of thinking and feeling, it seems to become a temporary, finite self. When it colours itself with sensation and perception, it seems to become a body and the world.

There is just God's infinite being assuming the appearance of all that exists without ever ceasing to be, to know and to love itself alone.

CHAPTER 4

NOTHING EXISTS, ONLY BEING IS

*This secret union takes place in the deepest centre
of the soul, which must be where God Himself dwells.*
SAINT TERESA OF AVILA

Just as there is no relationship between the physical space of the universe and the space that seems to be contained within a single building, for they are already the same space, so there is no relationship between God's infinite being and the temporary, finite self that we seem to be, for they are already the same being.

The person that we seem to be and the being that we truly are are one and the same. The actor John Smith, and the character he plays, King Lear, are identical. In both cases, the former is simply a temporary, illusory limitation of the latter.

Therefore, there is no question of an individual either being separated from or united with God's being. This understanding is expressed in the Vedantic tradition as *Ayam Atma Brahma:* the individual self and the ultimate reality of the universe are one and the same. In the

Christian tradition, 'I and my Father are one'.* In the Sufi tradition, 'Whosoever knows their self, knows their Lord'.†

As a compassionate concession to the person we seem to be, many traditions prescribe a method, practice or discipline whereby we may be united with God's being. One might argue that such methods validate and perpetuate the apparently separate self who undertakes them and are, as such, counterproductive. Or one might argue that such practices are the highest endeavour on which an individual can embark, placing the individual in the right relationship to God, and thus preparing it for its final dissolution in God's being. As the Sufi Bayazid Bastami said, 'What we speak of here cannot be found by seeking, and yet only seekers find it'.††

Such practices take us to the threshold. They empty the self of the self. This is all we can do. From there, God's being takes us into itself.

* * *

* The Gospel of John, 10:30.
† Twinch *op. cit.*
†† Quoted in James Fadiman and Robert Frager, *Essential Sufism* (Harper-Collins, 1997).

What does this seeking consist of?

Although there is only one infinite, indivisible being, we seem to be separate, limited individuals, and so we feel incomplete, lacking, dissatisfied and cut off from others. Hence, sorrow and conflict are the inevitable consequences of the belief in separation.

To re-establish the unity of being, the apparent individual undertakes a process which could be divided into two parts: interior and exterior prayer.

In interior prayer, we withdraw from the content of experience and sink into the sanctuary of the heart.

The Gospel of Saint Matthew describes it this way: 'When thou prayest, enter into thy closet, and when thou hast shut thy door, pray to thy Father, who is in secret'.* To 'shut thy door' is to turn away from sense perception through which the mind flows outwards into the world. To 'enter into thy closet' is to turn within and give our love and attention to the fact of simply being. It is the sinking of the mind into the heart. It is to enter the shrine of the heart in which the altar 'I am' stands. It is to rest in being, as being.

* The Gospel of Matthew, 6:6.

THE HEART OF PRAYER

Jesus was teaching his disciples self-abidance, the essence of prayer.

This subsidence of the mind into the heart is the surrendering of the separate self to God's presence. As the Indian sage Ramana Maharshi said, 'One who is steadily established in their being, giving not the slightest room for the arising of any thought, alone is surrendering their self to God'.*

* * *

Exterior prayer is the practice we undertake when we come out of our closet and return to the world. It is the prayer we carry out in the midst of our activities and relationships, as opposed to the interior prayer which we undertake in the privacy of the heart.

When Jesus said, 'When thou prayest, enter into thy closet, and when thou hast shut thy door, pray to thy Father, who is in secret', he might have continued with another verse: 'When thou prayest, open thy door, come out of thy closet, and see God's infinite being, which does not only lie in secret *behind* the world but manifests itself *as* the world'.

* Attributed to Ramana Maharshi.

In the Gospel of Thomas, Jesus says, 'If they ask you what is the sign of the Father in you, tell them it is a movement and a rest'.* This rest is the essence of our inner experience. It is the silence of the heart. The movement is our outer experience, the myriad changing forms that the one changeless being assumes without ever ceasing to be itself.

Form is emptiness in motion; emptiness is form at rest.

Praise is prayer in movement; prayer is praise in silence.

In exterior prayer, we come out of the closet of the heart and return to the world. Prayer ceases to be something special that we do at certain times. Our thoughts, feelings, sensations, perceptions, activities and relationships become prayers made manifest. Our life becomes a prayer of praise and thanksgiving.

There is no longer any question of having to guard the candle in the wind, because the world has caught fire and is ablaze with God's being. We may still choose, from time to time, to enter our closet and rest in being, as being, but this would not be any different from our everyday life in the world. It is simply a different mode of the same experience.

* The Gospel of Thomas, 50:3.

*   *   *

What does exterior prayer consist of? It is not so much something we do, as it is a felt understanding that gradually pervades and ultimately outshines our experience in the world.

Being is formless and, as such, there is nothing finite within it. It is infinite. Having nothing in itself other than itself, it is indivisible. It is one. Whatever emerges out of being – whatever exists – has a name and a form, which distinguishes it from all other names and forms. So whatever exists is limited, temporary and finite, although its limitation pertains only to its name and form, not to its reality, which remains whole, undivided and infinite.

This is what William Blake meant when he said, 'If the doors of perception were cleansed every thing will appear to man as it is, Infinite'.* When we see through the limitations that sense perception superimposes on reality, it is revealed as it is – infinite. It is this unlimited, formless, indivisible reality or being that manifests itself as the multiplicity and diversity of objects and selves. The one appears as the many.

* From *The Marriage of Heaven and Hell*, in *The Complete Poetry & Prose of William Blake* (Anchor, revised edition, 1982).

The screen is one thing – transparent, empty, indivisible. The movie appears to be many things – people, animals, objects. As such, the movie is in the same relationship to the screen as existence is to being.

Let us upgrade our analogy of the screen and the movie to space and a hologram. The empty, unlimited, indivisible space represents being, and the hologram is an appearance of the multiplicity and diversity which the empty space assumes.

Just as no people, animals or things ever really emerge out of the space of the hologram with their own independent existence, so no person, animal or thing ever emerges out of infinite being with an independent reality of its own.

Just as the characters and objects in a movie are colourings of the screen, just as the people and things in a hologram are appearances of the space, so everything and everyone is an appearance of God's infinite being. The universe derives its reality from God's infinite being and its appearance from the faculties of sense perception through which it is perceived. As William Wordsworth suggests, we half create, half perceive the world.

* * *

There are no things! Nothing exists! Only God's being truly is.

Nothing ever stands out from being with a discrete and independent existence. There is only God's being, refracting itself within itself, appearing as a multiplicity and diversity without ever ceasing to be itself.

The phrase *La ilaha illallah*, which stands at the heart of the Islamic tradition, and which has been so misunderstood, is traditionally translated as, 'There is no god but God'. If properly understood, this phrase distils thousands of years of spiritual investigation, practice and understanding into a few simple words.

Such phrases are like seeds planted in our minds and watered with our contemplation. In time, they grow within us, their meaning unfolding in our minds and delivering their nectar to our hearts. Such is the power of language.

A more contemporary translation of this phrase would be, 'Nothing exists; only being is'. Nothing has a reality or an identity of its own. Everyone and everything borrows its apparent reality from that which truly is, God's infinite, indivisible, immutable being.

This understanding is the foundation not only of the great religious and spiritual traditions but of both the Western and Eastern philosophical traditions. The fifth-century BCE Greek philosopher Parmenides considered that which *is* to be uncaused, unchanging, permanent and indestructible. In the Bhagavad Gita it says, 'That which is never ceases to be. That which is not never comes into existence.'*

That which is – eternal, infinite being – never commences or ceases to be, never appears or disappears. Beginning and ending require time. Appearance and disappearance require space. Time and space are not inherent in reality. They are modes of knowledge and perception, respectively. Time and space are how the one eternal, infinite reality appears when it is known through the localised perspective of a finite mind. The finite mind, through its activities of thought and perception, superimposes its own limitations on reality, thus rendering the infinite finite.

Others, recognising that it is impossible to describe reality with words that have evolved to describe its apparent parts,

* The Bhagavad Gita, 2:16.

use language in a way that attempts to confound our reasoning faculties, precipitating in us a direct recognition of reality itself.

'Before Abraham was, I am.'* That which is, eternally is. That which is not – people, animals and objects – never comes into existence. They never stand out from the background of being with their own independent reality. They are simply a colouring of that which truly is.

There is no creation. There are no things! There is the *appearance* of things.

What is it that is appearing? God's infinite, formless, unchanging being.

As Balyani said, 'You do not see God as having ever created anything, but as being every day in a different configuration which sometimes reveals Him and sometimes conceals Him'.†

*   *   *

Objects only seem to exist from the localised perspective of a finite mind. It is God's infinite, self-aware being that

* The Gospel of John, 8:59.
† Twinch *op. cit.*

64

localises itself in the form of each of our minds, from whose perspective its own activity appears as the universe.

If the appearance of objects is only such from the localised perspective of a separate subject of experience, what is God's direct experience? It must be the only true knowledge there is – that knowledge which is not mediated through the limitations of a finite mind. What is God's experience of itself prior to its apparent localisation in the form of a finite mind?

To see anything, we must stand apart from it. For this reason, the eyes cannot see themselves. Likewise, to know anything, we must stand apart from the object or experience that is known as a separate subject or knower. It is only from the apparent distance of a separate subject that an object or experience may be known.

However, God cannot stand apart from itself. There is no time or space in God's being and, therefore, no dimension in which it might stand apart from itself and know itself from a distance.

God's knowledge of itself is an utterly unique knowledge. God knows itself simply by being itself.

God's knowledge of itself – absolute knowledge – is unknown to the mind, which can only know in subject–object relationship. As Meister Eckhart said, 'Since it is God's nature not to be identical to anything other than itself, we must come to the state of being nothing in order to be one with God's nature. It is, therefore, in unknowing that the mind comes closest to God.'*

Therefore, from God's point of view we cannot even say there is the appearance of things. There is only the appearance of things from the perspective of the finite mind which is *itself* an appearance. The world is an illusion known only by the illusory finite mind.

Only God's infinite being eternally is, being only itself, knowing only itself. Thus, in God's knowledge of itself, there is no knowledge and no activity.

This absence of the knowledge of anything other than itself is the experience referred to as love. Love is, as such, the very nature of God. Thus, whenever we experience love in relationship, we are experiencing God's presence shining through the appearance of otherness.

The same experience in relationship to things is referred to as beauty. Thus, beauty is the very nature of God. In the

* Walshe *op. cit.*

experience of beauty, the object ceases to be an object and shines with its reality.

In God's knowledge of itself, there is no movement or activity. Thus, when we are still, we come closest to God's being. 'Be still and Know that I am God'.* Or, as Meister Eckhart said, 'Nothing in all creation is so like God as stillness'.†

* * *

The mind cannot grasp this understanding but can be in-formed by it. This understanding is like a crack in the world. A mind that has been touched by it is never the same again.

Initially, meditation or prayer could be described as the sinking of the mind into the heart of being. Later it could be considered the suffusing of the mind with the radiance of the heart.

This understanding is not taken in from the outside. It is conceived in the heart and spreads to all realms of our objective experience, informing our thoughts with its in-nate intelligence, infusing our feelings with its intrinsic

---

* Book of Psalms, 46:10.
† Walshe *op. cit.*

love and pervading our perceptions with its inherent beauty.

The world ceases to veil God's being but shines with it, as it.

At my first boarding school, we sang the same hymn in chapel every Sunday evening. I always associate it with the homesickness I felt there but later realised it was connected to a deeper homesickness – a nostalgia to return to the true home in the depths of my being. It awakened my early childhood intuition that the world is God's dream, a vision to which I longed to return.

> God be in my head and in my understanding.
> God be in my eyes and in my looking.
> God be in my mouth and in my speaking.
> God be in my heart and in my thinking.
> God be at my end and at my departing.*

* * *

Somebody once said, 'When the journey to God comes to an end, the journey in God begins'. For the journey *to* God,

* The Sarum Prayer, anonymous.

we turn away from thinking and perceiving, while the journey *in* God requires that we turn back and recognise that we share our being with everyone and everything.

Truly, there is no 'we' to share our being. The characters and objects in a movie do not share the screen, because there are no real characters or objects either to share or not to share it. There is just the one screen appearing as many but never ceasing to be itself.

To suggest that people and things share their being is a concession to their apparent existence. It is a legitimate concession at a certain stage of understanding, but eventually it must be abandoned.

Being is one infinite and indivisible whole from which all people and things borrow their apparent existence. Being is perfect, whole and complete, to which nothing can be added and from which nothing can be removed.

Where would such a thing come from? From non-being? Where would such a thing go when it disappeared? Into non-being? How could that which is emerge from that which is not? What is the status of 'that which is not' apart from an abstract idea?

*　*　*

To suggest that the world is a distraction from God's being is to credit the world with an existence of its own that subsequently has the power to veil God's being. It is like suggesting that a movie veils the screen. To do so, the movie would have to be something other than the screen.

If the world veils God's being, it would have to be something other than God's being, in which case God's being would not be infinite. God would not be God.

To suggest that the world is a distraction from God's being is a legitimate concession to one whose attention is so absorbed in the content of experience as to have overlooked its reality. For that one, it is necessary to turn away temporarily from the world to recognise God's being in and as their very own self.

Eventually it is necessary to turn around again and see the world, which once seemed to veil God's being, shining in and as that very being. The world is no longer seen as a distraction that veils or eclipses God's being but is understood instead to shine with it. As the Sufis say, 'Wherever you look, there is the face of God'.

The world is not *what* we see; it is *the way* we see. If we give the illusory world permission to veil God's infinite being, then it will seem to do so. If we withdraw that permission, the world which once seemed to veil God's being is now seen and felt to shine with it, as it.

*   *   *

A mind that is accustomed to resting in God's presence, subsiding in the heart and losing its limitations, is gradually and progressively washed clean of the dualising concepts that divide experience into self and other, mind and matter, God and the world. When such a mind rises again out of the heart of being, it emerges with insight, inspiration, understanding and creativity.

First our being is lost in the world; then our being returns to itself and, divested of the limitations that it borrows from the content of experience, stands revealed as God's being; then the world is lost in God's being.

This last step is referred to in the Tantric tradition of Kashmir Shaivism as 'devouring the world'. In the Christian tradition, these three steps are enshrined in the Crucifixion, the Resurrection and the Transfiguration. In the Crucifixion, individual being loses itself in God's being; in the

71

Resurrection, God's being shines as the 'I am' in each of us; and in the Transfiguration, God's being so utterly pervades and infuses the world that it is seen and felt to shine in and as God's being alone.

William Blake imagined explaining this understanding to a friend: ' "What", it will be Questioned, "When the Sun rises, do you not see a round disk of fire somewhat like a Guinea?" Oh no, no, I see an innumerable company of the Heavenly host crying, "Holy, Holy, Holy is the Lord God Almighty".'*

For one whose mind is steeped in God's presence, fewer and fewer thoughts and feelings arise on behalf of a temporary, finite, separate self. The activities and relationships in which we previously engaged in the service of such a self gradually leave us. Such a mind no longer serves the individual; it becomes impersonal. When turned inwards, it rests in its innate peace. When turned outwards, its purpose is to share, communicate or celebrate the qualities that are the nature of being: peace, joy, love. Prayer and praise.

Interior prayer is the pathway we take from 'I am something' to 'I am nothing'. Exterior prayer is the pathway

---

* A Vision of the Last Judgment' (c. 1810), *Selected Poems from William Blake*, edited by P. H. Butter (Everyman, 1982).

from 'I am nothing' to 'I am everything'. The former is the journey to God, the latter the journey in God. The former is the Crucifixion and Resurrection, the latter the Transfiguration, the outshining of the world in the radiance of God's being.

These two aspects of prayer were expressed by Shantananda Saraswati in this way:

> If you begin to be what you are, you will realise everything, but to begin to be what you are, you must come out of what you are not. You are not those thoughts which are turning, turning in your mind; you are not those changing feelings; you are not the different decisions you make and the different wills you have; you are not the separate ego. Well then, what are you? You will find when you have come out of what you are not, that the ripple on the water is whispering to you 'I am That', the birds in the trees are singing to you 'I am That', the moon and the stars are shining beacons to you 'I am That'. You are in everything in the world and everything in the world is reflected in you, and at the same time you are That – everything.*

* *Good Company: An Anthology of Sayings, Stories and Answers by His Holiness Shantanand Saraswati 1961–1985* (The Study Society, 1987).

CHAPTER 5

THE DARK NIGHT OF THE SOUL

In the dark night of the soul, bright flows the river of God.
SAINT JOHN OF THE CROSS

The separate self or ego is a mixture of infinite being plus the content of experience – thoughts, images, feelings, sensations, activities and relationships. Consequently, 'I am' becomes, or seems to become, 'I am this' or 'I am that'.

This mixture of our essential self with the qualities of experience creates the illusion of a separate self, a being apart from God's being. However, sometimes something happens in our life that fractures this narrative – the breakup of a relationship, the death of a loved one, financial loss, ill health – and the separate self or ego around whom the narrative is woven feels its existence threatened. The separate self sustains its illusory existence by identification with a person, group, religion, ideal, status, achievement and so on, and in the absence of anything or anyone to identify with, it cannot stand.

Feeling the emptiness of everything in which they have previously invested their desire for security and happiness, many turn to a religious or spiritual tradition. Indeed, these teachings do help some people to lead a more meaningful life, sustaining them for many years.

However, sometimes the trust we previously invested in our spiritual teaching or teacher and, for those on a devotional path, our faith in God, is removed from us. At this point, we have exhausted all possibilities. There is simply nowhere left to turn.

This is what Saint John of the Cross called the 'dark night of the soul', a desert in which one feels that everything has been taken away, most especially the presence of God.

In this existential crisis, the mind is faced with its utter inability to do anything about its current predicament. It cannot reach for consolation, even from God. 'My God, my God, why hast Thou forsaken me?'* is the familiar feeling of one who is experiencing this dark night of the soul.

* The Gospel of Matthew, 27:46.

Every possible avenue of escape and consolation has been withdrawn. Our sorrow is both unbearable and unavoidable. There is nowhere to turn, nothing to do. There are no solutions, no practices, no comforting ideas, no prospect of future happiness.

In the dark night of the soul, one must sit without expectation. In the words of T. S. Eliot, 'I said to my soul, "Be still and wait without hope, for hope would always be hope for the wrong thing. Wait without love, for love would always be love for the wrong thing".'* We sit without regret or expectation. Regret takes us into the past, expectation into the future.

However, it is possible that the dark night of the soul may lead not to despair but to surrender, for even this darkness is pervaded by the experience of being. If I am depressed, I am present there; if I am lonely, I am present there; if I am anxious, I am present there.

Even in this dark night of the soul, being shines. Being is like the sun: it cannot be extinguished. It shines brightly even in the darkest places.

* From 'East Coker', *Four Quartets* (Harcourt, 1941).

This is what Meister Eckhart referred to when he said, 'Truly it is in the darkness that one finds the light, so when we are in sorrow then this light is nearest of all to us'.*

For the separate self, this darkness, including even the absence of any hope or possibility of redemption, is the ultimate loss. But for one on a spiritual path, it is the removal of everything that perpetuates the sense of our self as a being apart from God's being. 'When I am able to establish myself in nothing and nothing in myself, uprooting and casting out what is in me, then I can pass into the naked being of God, which is the naked being of the Spirit.'†

When all possible consolations are removed and everything that is not essential to us is stripped away, it feels like darkness to the mind. The ego is a mixture of our essential being with the qualities of experience, therefore, in the dark night of the soul, when everything in which we have invested our identity has been removed, the ego feels like it is dying. It becomes, as Meister Eckhart says, like nothing. All that remains of it is the light of God's being.

* Walshe *op. cit.*
† Walshe *op. cit.*

In this darkness, the pure, unqualified 'I am' emerges from behind its disguise of 'I am this' or 'I am that'.

God's presence begins to shine in and as our very own being.

*   *   *

The way of devotion, Bhakti Yoga, is really the same path as the way of knowledge, Jnana Yoga. Only in the early stages of these two practices – self-surrender and self-enquiry – do they seem to differ. However, the more deeply we go into them, the more they converge and are recognised to be the same path, albeit formulated in different ways.

Brother Lawrence said, 'Let us occupy ourselves entirely knowing God. The more we know him, the more we will desire to know him. As love increases with knowledge, the more we know God, the more we truly love Him.'* As our knowledge of the nature of being increases, so our love of simply being deepens.

God is our very own being. Therefore, the ultimate devotion – the practice of the presence of God – is simply to

---

* *The Practice of the Presence of God: The Original 17th Century Letters and Conversations of Brother Lawrence* (Xulon Press, 2007).

abide in and as inherently peaceful and unconditionally fulfilled being.

To devote ourself to a God outside ourself depends upon the existence of a self apart from God. Although this form of dualistic devotion curtails the separate self, and thus prepares it for the ultimate surrender – abiding in and as being – it ultimately perpetuates it. The object of our longing depends upon the existence of a separate self as the subject of that longing. As long as the object persists, the subject continues. As long as the beloved endures, the devotee remains.

God lies at the source of our longing; it can never be an object of our longing. Let go of the object of your longing and allow yourself, the subject of your longing, to subside into the love from which both arise: God's infinite being.

Many people develop a love for God who they conceive as separate and at an infinite distance from themselves. However, once it is realised that God is our very own being, then our love is redirected from God, who seems to be apart from ourself, to our very own being. As Ramana Maharshi said, 'To abide in and as simply being is the ultimate devotion to God'.*

* Attributed to Ramana Maharshi.

This directing of our love towards our innermost being – God's being – is felt by the individual as something that we *do* or *practise*. In fact, it is the pull of the grace of God attracting the apparently separate self back into itself.

What feels like an effort to the individual is the gravitational pull of our own being, God's being, on its own contracted, limited form, the separate self or ego.

What we experience as the search for happiness is happiness searching for us. As Hafiz said, 'Ever since happiness heard your name, it has been running through the streets trying to find you'.*

*   *   *

Initially, we seem to take a step towards God, but in time, we feel that we are drawn by the gravitational pull of God's presence. This is what Brother Lawrence was referring to when he said, 'In order to form a habit of communing with God continually and committing everything we do to him, we must, at first, make a special effort. After a while,

* From 'Several Times in the Last Week', *I Heard God Laughing: Renderings of Hafiz*, translated by Daniel Ladinsky (Penguin Books, 2006).

we find that his love inwardly inspires us to do all things for him effortlessly.'*

As objective experience loses its capacity to take us away from our self, God's being, we begin to feel God's presence pulling us into the heart, attracting us into itself. This is the power of grace which is always operating within us. It is the still, small voice that constantly whispers, 'Turn round, come back to me. I am your home and refuge; I am your self.'

Self-surrender is simply to give up the belief and feeling that we are separate from or other than God's infinite being. It is to remain as we are, without allowing our being to be qualified by the content of experience. That is the love of God.

However, it would be a mistake to conclude that God's being is only the essence of each of us and not the essence of the world. God's being is not only that from which we derive our being; it is that from which the world borrows its apparent existence.

The mind's activity is the form in which the one appears as the many. Having refracted itself into an apparent multiplicity

* *The Practice of the Presence of God: The Original 17th Century Letters and Conversations of Brother Lawrence* (Xulon Press, 2007).

and diversity of objects and selves, it experiences – in the form of one of those selves – sorrow on the inside and conflict on the outside. These are the inevitable consequence of infinite being's apparent fragmentation of itself into individual beings and things.

However, turning back, it ceases to fragment itself through the activities of thinking and perceiving, and returns to its natural condition of wholeness, perfection and peace. God comes into the place of our self.

In the words of Meister Eckhart, 'Whoever possesses God in their being has Him in a divine manner, and He shines out to them in all things; for them all things taste of God and in all things it is God's image that they see'.* That is, ultimately, there are no things. There is just God's infinite being clothed in name and form, appearing as things without ever ceasing to be itself.

Again, Meister Eckhart: 'If the soul is to know God it must forget itself and lose itself, for as long as it contemplates self, it cannot contemplate God. When it has lost itself and everything in God, it finds itself again in God when it attains to the knowledge of Him, and it

* Walshe *op. cit.*

83

finds also everything which it had abandoned complete in God.'*

* * *

Longing is to the heart what seeking is to the mind. Seeking is the directing of awareness towards an object; longing is the directing of love towards the beloved. The ultimate object towards which we direct our love is God.

Initially, on the path of devotion, God is considered to be separate and at a distance from ourself. Hence, the traditional dualistic practices of devotion. However, just as the highest form of meditation – simply being – does not involve the directing or focusing of attention, but rather the sinking or relaxing of attention into the source of awareness from which it arises, so the ultimate prayer is not a movement or a reaching of our longing towards God, but a relaxing or subsiding of our longing into the source of love from which it originates.

Just as we cannot pay attention *to* awareness, we pay attention *from* awareness; likewise, God's being lies at the

* Walshe *op. cit.*

84

source of our longing and can never be an *object* of our longing.

Our longing is God's love directed towards the content of experience. When our longing is divested of its object, it sinks into its source and stands revealed as God's love.

As such, the ultimate devotion or surrender to God is to divest our longing of its object, the beloved, and to allow our longing to subside back into the love from which it arises. As Meister Eckhart said, 'The love by which we love God is the very same love with which God has first loved us'.*

Only awareness is aware and, therefore, awareness can only be known by itself. Likewise, God is love and, therefore, God can only be loved by itself, not by a person.

In love we stand as God; in longing we stand as the person. Let your longing come to rest in this understanding.

*   *   *

If the way of negation, the Via Negativa, culminates in the understanding that God is nothing – not a thing – then the

* Walshe *op. cit.*

way of affirmation, the Via Positiva, culminates in the understanding that God is everything.

The way of negation is the way of prayer or surrender; the way of affirmation is the way of praise or love. In prayer, we sink into the depths of being; in love, we embrace everyone and everything as that being.

These two – prayer or surrender and praise or love – are not really two different conditions. The only condition is God's being.

In prayer, we rest in God's being; in praise, we celebrate God's being.

In sorrow, we long for God; in joy, we love God.

In our longing, God's being is concealed; in love, God's being is revealed.

There is only love or the veiling of love but never its absence. If love is concealed, we live in a state of longing; if love is revealed, we live in a state of praise.

Praise doesn't necessarily imply verbal praise. It could take the form of many kinds of activity or relationship in which the unity of being is expressed, celebrated and shared, and in which the mind and body become the servants of love and understanding.

In time, the distinction between sorrow and happiness begins to blur. They are no longer felt as opposites. In sorrow, we hear God's call; in joy, we listen to God's song. Just like a mother who hears her infant crying one moment and laughing another, loving it equally in both cases, so we feel and love God's presence equally in sorrow and joy.

Our longing and our joy – the minor and major keys of the same song – are outshone in God's being.

* * *

Meister Eckhart said, 'To be receptive to the highest truth and to live therein, a person must be without before and after, untrammelled by all their actions or by anything they have ever perceived or experienced, empty and free, receiving the divine gift in the eternal now, and bearing it back unhindered in the light of the same with praise and thanksgiving'.*

* My rendition of Maurice O'C. Walshe's translation from *The Complete Mystical Works of Meister Eckhart* (Herder & Herder, 2010).

Sooner or later, all spiritual and religious traditions culminate in a single recognition: there is no pathway from the person we seem to be to the being we essentially are. There is no distance from our self to our self. There is no practice that can take us from the sense of being an individual to God's infinite being, because the former is simply an apparent limitation of the latter.

Our previous practice, which involved effort on the horizontal dimension of time, is replaced by sinking into the vertical dimension of being. The intersection of these two dimensions is the 'now'. From the individual's perspective, now is considered a moment in time; from being's perspective, now is eternity.

Likewise, the horizontal dimension of time and the vertical dimension of being intersect in the name 'I'. In other words, 'I' is the name that the individual gives to itself, and 'I' is the name that being would give to itself if it could speak. The 'I' that stands at the heart of the individual is the 'I' of God's infinite being. Sound the name 'I' once and allow it to draw you into the innermost sanctuary of the heart, pure being.

If we were to ask being, prior to the arising of experience, 'What is your experience of yourself?', it would remain silent.

That would be the most honest response. If pressed, as a concession to the one who asks, pure being would respond, 'In my own experience of myself, there is nothing other than myself. I simply am.'

The words 'I am' refer directly to being's experience of itself, our knowledge of our self, God's knowledge of itself.

*　　*　　*

If we were to ask being, 'Do you know any limitation in yourself?', it would respond, 'There is nothing in myself other than myself. Therefore, I know nothing of limitation, but as a concession to your question and with reference to the limited content of experience, I am unlimited.' That is, the idea that being is unlimited or infinite is only a concession to our belief in limited or finite things. Being knows nothing of such things and, therefore, has no need to define itself in reference to them. But as a concession to our belief in limited, finite things, being consents to say of itself, 'I am unlimited or infinite'.

If we were to ask being, 'Do you have any experience of the beginning or ending of yourself?', being would say, 'In my own experience of myself, I have no knowledge of starting or stopping, appearing or disappearing, birth or death. I eternally am.'

If we were to ask being, 'Do you ever lack anything?', it would respond, 'In my own experience of myself, I am whole, indivisible, perfect and complete. Everything that exists, or seems to exist, borrows its being from me. The sense of lack is only for one of the apparent parts. Thus, happiness is my nature.'

If we were to ask being, 'Do you have any desires?', being would respond, 'I am that in which all desires come to rest'. At this point, being might say, 'Given that all your desires are destined to return to me, why not stay with me to begin with? Why travel the world in search of home? It is not necessary to do anything in order to be.'

If we were to ask being, 'What do you know of people and things?', it would respond, 'Everyone and everything derives its apparent existence from me. It is I who appear as people and things without ever ceasing to be myself. People and things are only such from the perspective of a person. In my own experience of myself, there is only myself. I know nothing of otherness. Thus, my nature is love.'

Being would then say, 'When you experience love, it is I who am experiencing myself in you. You do not exist as yourself. Your being is my being. You only seem to exist in your own mistaken view of yourself. I am the self of yourself. It is from me that you derive your sense of yourself. Only you have allowed me to become mixed with the content of experience and thus believe yourself to be temporary, finite and limited. I am the infinite "I", the only "I" there is. It is through me that you know yourself as yourself. It is in and through me that you seem to have your own existence. You borrow your existence from my being.'

*   *   *

Divested of 'before and after', we stand empty and free in the eternal now, in naked being, utterly intimate, yet impersonal and infinite.

Rumi said, 'Be like melting snow, wash yourself of yourself'.* This self-emptying, self-forgetting, is the highest form of devotion. It is the practice of the presence of God. It is the place at which our longing for happiness turns into our love of simply being, our love of God.

If there is the slightest feeling of boredom, irritation or lack in meditation or prayer, it is because we have left the eternal now and followed thought into the past or future.

* *The Essential Rumi*, translated by Coleman Barks (HarperOne, 2004).

Therein lies our sorrow. We think our sorrow exists in the now and that we escape from it into the past and future, but the opposite is true. Our sorrow exists only in reference to the past and future. It cannot stand in the now.

Make the now your refuge. It is the place of peace.

*   *   *

Why do so many traditions encourage the worship of an external God? As a compassionate concession to the separate self that we seem to be. This is legitimate for one who is devoted to God outside themselves. We should not take that away from them but allow the impulse towards God to run its course. In time, we begin to intuit that the God we previously sought outside ourself lives as our very own being.

Imagine that the actor John Smith is so deeply involved in the role of King Lear that he believes he *is* King Lear. As a compassionate concession, his friend says to him, 'Imagine a loving being called John Smith who loves you unconditionally. Direct your love and devotion to him.'

Believing himself to be King Lear, he imagines John Smith to be someone outside himself. It is only in reference to that belief that his friend says to him, 'Devote yourself to a personal God called John Smith'.

Later, through devotion to John Smith, King Lear's sense of himself begins to diminish, and he begins to intuit that John Smith is, in fact, the very essence of himself.

Likewise, in our experience there is what the Old Testament refers to as a 'conversion', a turning around. We begin to understand and feel that the God we previously sought outside ourself, at an infinite distance from ourself, is our very own being.

Either gradually or suddenly, there is the recognition that we are that for which we long. In words attributed to Lalla, the fourteenth-century mystic and poet from the Kashmir Shaivite tradition, 'I have travelled a long way seeking God, but when I finally gave up and turned back, there He was, within me'.

CHAPTER 6

THE ONE

It is because there is nothing in the One that all things are from it.

PLOTINUS

Imagine removing all your thoughts. Thoughts are continually appearing, existing briefly and vanishing of their own accord, so it is not difficult to imagine removing the current thought and not replacing it with another.

Imagine removing all images from your experience. Simply imagine experiencing yourself in the absence of thoughts and images.

Imagine removing your memories. No memory is essential to us; they all appear and disappear. Stay with your experience of yourself in the absence of memories.

In the absence of thought, there is no knowledge of the future; in the absence of memory, there is no knowledge of the past. So we simply find ourself present now – not now, a moment in time, for without reference to thought or memory there is no experience of time, but the ever-present, eternal now. Without reference to the future, there is no anxiety or fear. Without reference to the past, there is no sorrow, regret, shame or guilt.

Imagine removing your feelings and simply remain as yourself. We are removing those elements of our experience that are not essential to us.

Allow the experience of the body to come to your attention. Without reference to thoughts, images or memory, we have no knowledge or experience of either having or being a body. There are just sensations – not sensations *of* a body but just raw, unnameable sensations. Imagine removing all your sensations. Sensations appear and then vanish, so none are essential to us. Remain with your experience of yourself.

Imagine removing all your perceptions of the world. None are essential to us. They pass through us without leaving a trace on us. Simply be as you are in the absence of all perceptions.

Imagine removing all your activities. None are essential to us. Simply remain as you are in the absence of all activities. Imagine removing all your relationships. None are essential to us and, therefore, cannot be what we essentially are. Simply remain as you are in the absence of relationship.

*   *   *

All that remains when thoughts, images, feelings, sensations, perceptions, activities and relationships have been removed from us is the experience of simply being, the awareness of being. The awareness of being cannot be removed from us. It is our essential, irreducible self.

Our being cannot legitimately be named and yet all our names refer to it. It has no form but is present – nameless, formless being, God's infinite being.

If infinite being were to give itself a name, it would call itself 'I', for 'I' is the name that anything that knows itself gives to itself. We know our own being – that is, our being knows itself – before it knows any other thing. Therefore, the name 'I' is the first form of God in the finite mind. It is the divine name.

As long as nothing is added to 'I', it refers directly to God's infinite being, but when 'I' is qualified by experience, it acquires a name and form. Infinite being seems to become a temporary, finite self. Therefore, 'I' is the portal through which infinite being passes out of eternity into time, and the same portal through which the separate self passes, in the opposite direction, out of time into eternity.

All experience is pervaded by 'I'. Let every experience take you to 'I', and from 'I' to God's being.

Simply abide as that.

*　　*　　*

The mind refers to God's being as infinite because it compares it with the finite things that it seems to know, but in being's experience of itself, there are no finite things. Therefore, there is nothing in itself to compare itself with, so it does not know itself as infinite. It is prior to and beyond the finite and the infinite.

Simply abide as that.

The finite mind refers to God's being as peace because it compares it to its own agitation, but in being's experience of itself, it knows no agitation and thus does not know itself as peace. It is prior to and beyond peace and agitation.

Simply abide as that.

In its own experience of itself, God's being knows no sorrow and, therefore, need not be conceptualised as happiness.

Simply abide as that.

In its own experience of itself, being knows no multiplicity or otherness and, therefore, need not be conceptualised with reference to an other as love, although it is that which shines in our hearts as the experience of love.

Simply abide as that.

In being's own experience of itself, there is no duality and, therefore, it knows nothing of non-duality – no subject or object, no person, no self, no world. It has nothing to become, nothing to renounce, nothing to attain, nothing to acquire. It knows no darkness and, therefore, no enlightenment. It seeks nothing, knows nothing, resists nothing, understands nothing.

Simply abide as that.

There is no distance from God's being to itself and, therefore, no room for a method, pathway, practice or discipline.

Simply abide as that.

In its own experience, there is no birth, no existence, no death. There is no creation and no destruction.

Simply abide as that.

*   *   *

Now allow the experience of thinking to reappear but remain abiding only as that. See that the experience of thinking appears within that and arises from that. When thinking begins, nothing new comes into existence; thinking is simply a movement of that. It is that, God's being, which assumes the activity of thinking without ever ceasing to be itself.

When a thought disappears, nothing real ceases to exist. Infinite being simply ceases assuming the activity of thinking and remains as itself. When the activity of thinking resumes, appearing as the next thought, God's being never becomes anything other than itself. It just remains as it is.

No thought comes into existence, no thought exists and no thought vanishes out of existence. There is just God's being, modulating itself in the form of thinking without ever ceasing to be itself.

Allow feeling to reappear but see that no actual emotion comes into existence. There is just God's being, modulating itself as the activity of feeling without ever ceasing to be itself. The feeling is empty, with no inherent existence of its own. It's just a self-assumed colouring of God's being. There is only that.

Allow the experience of sensing to reappear but don't allow a sensation, let alone a body, to come into existence. There is just God's being, modulating itself in the form of sensing, appearing to the mind as a body without ever ceasing to be itself.

All there is to the experience of the body is sensing, and sensing is the activity of the one infinite, immutable and indivisible reality – transparent, empty, luminous.

Allow the experience of seeing, hearing, touching, tasting and smelling to reappear, but don't let a world come into existence. There is just the one infinite, unnameable reality, modulating itself in the form of the world without ever ceasing to be itself, appearing as a world only from the localised perspective of a finite mind.

Simply abide as that.

Understand the world as a movement of the one reality within itself, made only of itself, never becoming anything other than itself. Nothing other than God's being ever comes into existence. Nothing is created, nothing exists, nothing is destroyed.

As Meister Eckhart says, 'All that God asks you most pressingly is to go out of yourself, and let God be God in you. As long as I am this or that, or have this or that, I am not all things and I have not all things. Become pure until you neither are, nor have neither this or that. Then you are omnipresent and, being neither this nor that, are all things.'*

*   *   *

The non-dual understanding is the revelation of the oneness of reality, the unity of being, behind and within the multiplicity and diversity of appearances. This reality cannot ultimately be named or defined, because all names and definitions arise with reference to its apparent parts. However, as a concession to our desire to speak of it, it has been given numerous names: God, Allah, Brahman, the Buddha, the Tao, Consciousness, Spirit, Love and so on. In their wisdom and humility, the ancient masters of the Vedantic tradition simply referred to it as *advaita*, or 'not two', preferring to say what it is not rather than what it is, thus preventing it from being confined to the finite mind.

The non-dual teaching is the means by which we see through appearances to that one reality. In other words, the non-dual *understanding* is always the same understanding – the revelation of oneness – whilst the non-dual

* Walshe *op. cit.*

teaching varies: it is the means by which we approach this oneness.

Whether we give it a name or leave it unnamed, the teaching provides the means by which we may first recognise this one reality and subsequently lead a life that is consistent with and an expression of it.

*   *   *

If reality is one, why does it appear to be many? Because we perceive it through our sense perceptions – seeing, hearing, touching, tasting and smelling. These faculties refract and fragment the one reality, making it appear as a multiplicity and diversity of objects and selves. Through the act of perceiving, the one appears as the many, but at no point does a separate perceiver or a perceived world come into existence. No separate subject or object of experience ever 'stands out from' the one with its own independent existence. These are just temporary and apparent modulations of the one.

When we fall asleep and dream, our mind seems to localise itself within itself as an apparently separate subject of experience, from whose perspective it views itself as the dreamed world. Likewise, the one reality, assuming the activity of perceiving, seems to localise itself within itself as a separate subject of experience, from whose point of view it perceives itself as the many, without ever actually ceasing to be itself or knowing anything other than itself.

It is as though the one puts on a virtual reality headset made of thinking and perceiving and, as a result, views its own dimensionless being as an apparent multiplicity and diversity of objects and selves in time and space. Time and space, and the events and objects they contain, are not, as such, inherent in reality. They are simply how reality appears from the limited and localised perspective of a finite mind.

*   *   *

Thus, the world that we perceive is an illusion. However, I do not mean to imply that it is unreal. An illusion is not something that is unreal; it is something that is real but is not what it appears to be. What does the world appear to be? A multiplicity and diversity of objects and selves made of something other than God's infinite being. What is it really? The one infinite and indivisible reality, which shines as the amness of all selves and the isness of all things.

As a result of the illusory nature of the world, almost all religious and spiritual traditions suggest, in the early stages, that it is necessary to turn away from the content of experience in order to recognise the reality that lies behind it.

However, this turning away is a concession to the belief that the things we turn away from are real in their own right. In other words, early on in this investigation, the objects of experience we turn away from are considered to be *other than* the one reality. We make a distinction between the one reality and everything else. I am not my thoughts; I am that which is aware of them. I am not my feelings and perceptions; I am that which knows them.

Whilst this is a legitimate step, eventually we must abandon it. If there is only one reality, then *everything must be that*. What is there to turn away from and who would turn away from it? If there is only one, then the one must always only be knowing itself, for there is nothing in itself other than itself either to know or to be known. Therefore, in the later stages of our exploration, we need to turn towards the experience from which we previously turned away and recognise it not as a veiling of God's being but the shining of God's being.

Even that is not quite right. Who is the one who would turn away from or towards the content of experience if there is only one and for what reason? If there is only one, who or what is it that would seek happiness, enlightenment or God?

Any search would come from the feeling that something is missing, but there is nothing other than God's being to be absent, nor is there anything other than itself to be gained or acquired. How could the one practise anything, or make any effort or move towards some future state?

The place where it started would be itself; its practice, effort or discipline would be itself; and the place at which it arrived would be itself. It would not, therefore, have done anything or gone anywhere.

*   *   *

For the one there cannot be any creation, because if it were to create something, that creation would be other than itself. Something other than itself would be a second reality. There would be itself *and* its creation. Therefore, the one would no longer be one. And if the one's creation were identical to itself, then it cannot be said to have created anything.

The one never appears or begins, because anything that appears must appear or arise in something that precedes it.

If there were something prior to the one, out of which it could arise or appear, then there would be something other than it, and the one would not be one. God would not be God.

Likewise, the one never disappears or comes to an end, because it would have to disappear into something that was other than itself, which existed prior to and in the absence of itself. Whatever that is would have to be greater than the one, in order to accommodate it. This would render the one finite, limited and temporary, in which case the one would no longer be the one. God would no longer be God.

Thus, in its own experience of itself, the one knows nothing of appearance and disappearance, that is, it knows nothing of birth and death. Any birth would imply the coming into existence of something other than itself, which is already fully present, and death would imply the losing of a part of itself, thus becoming incomplete.

If something were to be born, from where would it come? If something were to die, where would it go? Given there is nothing other than the one from which something could arise or into which it could vanish, it knows nothing of birth or death. Birth and death are for appearances, not for the one reality.

*   *   *

In the one's own experience of itself, it is eternal, not ever-lasting in time, because from its perspective there is no time present in which it might last. If the one appeared and lasted in time, time would precede it and be greater than it, and the one would thus be a limited appearance within it. In the one's own experience of itself, it is eternal.

The one is ever-present, not everlasting. When we think of eternity, it appears as time. That is, the ever-present filtered through thought appears as the everlasting. The best the finite mind can do is to conceive of eternity as the present moment. The idea of a present moment is the finite mind's attempt to bring the eternal within its own narrow compass and reconcile its belief in time with the experience of eternity.

The present moment is, as such, the place where the finite and the infinite intersect. It is the place where the horizontal line of time and the vertical dimension of eternity touch one another, as symbolised by the cross. For this reason, the present moment is considered a portal for the mind through which it passes out of time into eternity.

Thus, for the one there cannot be any time, because time involves the passing away of that which is present or the coming into existence of that which is not present. If something were to pass away, then the one, which is fully present now, would be diminished by it. If anything were to come into existence, the one, which is fully present now, would be enhanced by it. If the one could be diminished or enhanced, it would not be complete, whole and perfect. Therefore, for the one there is no time; there is only eternity.

For the one there is no experience of space, because space implies distance, and for the one there is no distance between itself and itself. We cannot even say that the one is everywhere, because there is no 'everywhere' for it to pervade. The idea that the one is everywhere is a thorn that is used to remove the thorn – a provisional idea used to remove the belief that the one is *somewhere*, located in a particular person, place or thing. Having removed that idea, we should abandon the idea that the one is everywhere. The idea that the one is everywhere is as far as the mind can go. Beyond that it cannot venture.

All experience takes place 'here'. We never find the place we call 'there', for whenever we arrive 'over there', it is still always 'here'. The experience 'I am' always takes place here and now – not 'here', a place in space, or 'now', a moment in time, but here and now, the placeless place where I, infinite being, eternally am.

It is only something other than our self – other than God's being – that seems to take place then and there, in a particular place in space and moment in time. Like the now, the idea of 'here' is where the finite and the infinite intersect. For the mind, 'here' is a place in space. For the one, the same 'here' is its own dimensionless presence, the placeless place where 'I am', where God is.

*   *   *

For the one there is nothing lacking, because the one could only lack something other than itself. If there were something other than itself, then the one would not be one. For the one there is no imperfection, because there is nothing in itself other than itself out of which any imperfection could be made. Any imperfection would be like a white spot on a white page, which is no imperfection at all. Thus, the one is whole, perfect, complete.

For the one there is no sorrow, because sorrow implies resistance, and there is nothing in the one other than the one which could either resist or be resisted. This absence of resistance is the experience we know as happiness – unconditional happiness that knows no opposite and is not derived from the content of experience. It is simply the nature of the one.

Having nothing in itself other than itself, there can be no division within the one. Any division would exist only in its appearances, which could only be known from the limited perspective of a separate subject of experience. Any apparent division would be like a wall made of space appearing in space, or a white line drawn on a white page, dividing nothing from nothing. The one reality is, as such, indivisible.

Having nothing in itself other than itself, the one knows no other. If there were something other than the one, then the one would not be one. Thus, love – the absence of otherness – is its very nature. As such, the one knows nothing of separation and the conflict that inevitably attends it.

The experience of love is not, as such, an emotion that one person feels towards another; it is the absence of otherness or separation. It is the collapse of self and other. The experience of love is a revelation of reality filtering into our human experience. As a concession to the separate individual, we may say that love is the felt sense of our shared being. It is the one appearing as two. As such, friendship, which is an expression of love, is a vehicle for this understanding, a pathway in its own right.

For the one there are no objects, because an object would be something that exists in its own right. If there were objects as well as the one, then the one would not be one. In the absence of any objects, it cannot be said to be the subject, because there is nothing for it to be the subject of. Therefore, there is no subject–object relationship for the one. This is the experience of beauty.

* * *

For the one there is no desire, because desire is always a movement towards someone or something. There is nothing in the one, other than the one, towards which it could move. If the one were to move towards something, that thing would be itself. Its movement would be itself and the place from which it moved would be itself. Its movement would, therefore, be no movement at all, unless its desire were simply the pouring forth of itself within itself, in which case its desire would be creativity, the highest form of desire. In religious terms, praise and thanksgiving.

For the one there is no sickness, because any sickness would imply a state that was less than the perfection of itself. Any such state would be a second reality and, therefore, the one would not be one. This inherent absence of sickness, which is the nature of the one, is reflected in a human mind as its desire for a perfect state of health. Although informed by an intuition of its natural condition, which is free of any lack, disease or sickness, the mind projects this intuition onto the body, thereby conceiving of it in a way that is consistent with its own limitations. The ultimate healing is, as such, not a state of perfect health for the body; it is the recognition of the prior condition of wholeness which is the nature of the one.

The one does not know anything. Anything known would have a form and, therefore, a limit. Anything that is limited is a fragment or a part, and there are no parts in the one. Any fragment or part would only be known from the limited perspective of an apparently separate self. To know a thing or object, one must first stand apart from that thing as an apparently separate subject, just as the eyes can only see something that is at a distance from them. The one cannot stand apart from itself and, therefore, knows nothing.

This absence of knowledge seems like ignorance from the mind's perspective, but it is divine ignorance. It is a state in which there is no knowledge of things and yet the one shines all alone. It is true knowledge in which nothing is known. As Meister Eckhart said, 'Though it may be called a nescience, an unknowing, yet there is in it more than all knowing and understanding without it; for this unknowing lures and attracts you from all understood things, and from yourself as well'.*

Thus, the highest form of knowledge is to know nothing. Such knowledge is absolute. Anything that is known is relative to the mind through which it is known. However, all such knowledge is a refraction of the ultimate, absolute knowledge in which nothing is known.

It is for this reason that a mind that is touched by the absolute falls silent. With the mind silent, all that remains is simply being, God's being – the ultimate reality and the heart of prayer.

* Walshe *op. cit.*

Infinite, impersonal, intimate Being,

Who is the sole reality of all that exists,

Let your divine name, 'I', shine brightly
in our hearts at all times.

May we recognise our being as your being.

May our lives be an outpouring of
praise and thanksgiving,

Expressing your peace, your joy and your love
in all that we think and feel and do.

May we see you everywhere,
shining in and as the world.

Grant us the remembrance of your fullness,

From which our lives are derived and with
which they are sustained.

Forgive us those times when our actions betray
the overlooking of your presence,

And help us to forgive those who do not yet
know that their being is your being.

Keep our minds and hearts steady in
the knowledge of your presence,

Lest the belief in separation veil the peace
and love that you are.

For you alone are the reality of all that exists,

The one who performs all actions,

And the one whom we love in everyone
and everything, whether we know it or not.

Our only prayer, that you take us
into yourself, for all eternity.

Amen.*

---

* My rendering of the Lord's Prayer.

QUOTATION SOURCES

INVITATION
Plotinus, *Plotinus: Myth, Metaphor, and Philosophical Practice*, translated by Stephen R. L. Clark (University of Chicago Press, 2018)

CHAPTER ONE
Saint Catherine of Genoa, *The Life and Doctrine of Saint Catherine of Genoa* (Benediction Classics, 2012)

CHAPTER TWO
Joel Goldsmith, *The Mystical I* (Acropolis Books, 2018)

CHAPTER THREE
Meister Eckhart, *The Complete Mystical Works of Meister Eckhart*, translated by Maurice O'C. Walshe (Herder & Herder, 2010)

CHAPTER FOUR
Saint Teresa of Avila, *The Interior Castle, or the Mansions* (Antiquarius, 2020)

CHAPTER FIVE
Saint John of the Cross, *Dark Night of the Soul* (Whitaker House, 2017)

CHAPTER SIX

Plotinus, *The Essential Plotinus: Representative Treatises from the Enneads*, translated by Elmer O'Brien (New American Library, 1964)

THE ESSENCE OF MEDITATION SERIES

The Essence of Meditation Series presents meditations on the essential, non-dual understanding that lies at the heart of all the great religious and spiritual traditions. Taken from meditations led by Rupert Spira at his meetings and retreats, the simple, contemplative approach presented here encourages a clear seeing of one's experience, leading to an experiential understanding of the peace and causeless joy that are the true nature of our essential being.

Being Aware of Being Aware
The Essence of Meditation Series, Volume I

Being Myself
The Essence of Meditation Series, Volume II

The Heart of Prayer
The Essence of Meditation Series, Volume III

PUBLICATIONS BY RUPERT SPIRA

The Transparency of Things – Contemplating the Nature of Experience

Presence, Volume I – The Art of Peace and Happiness

Presence, Volume II – The Intimacy of All Experience

The Ashes of Love – Sayings on the Essence of Non-Duality

The Light of Pure Knowing
– Thirty Meditations on the Essence of Non-Duality

Transparent Body, Luminous World
– The Tantric Yoga of Sensation and Perception

The Nature of Consciousness – Essays on the Unity of Mind and Matter

A Meditation on I Am

The Essential Self – Three Meditations

You Are the Happiness You Seek – Uncovering the Awareness of Being

Naked, Self-Aware Being – A Seven-Day Retreat in New York

www.rupertspira.com